Air Fryer Best Recipes

Healthy and Tasty Meat Recipes for Air Fryer Diet

Franck McMillan

TABLE OF CONTENT

this book has been derived from various sources. Please consult a licensed professional before attempting any techniques outlined in this book.

By reading this document, the reader agrees that under no circumstances is the author responsible for any losses, direct or indirect, which are incurred as a result of the use of information contained within this document, including, but not limited to, — errors, omissions, or inaccuracies.

Banana and Walnut Cake

Preparation Time:10 minutes

Cooking Time: 25 minutes

Servings: 6

Ingredients:

- 1-pound (454g) bananas, mashed
- 8ounces (227g) flour
- 6ounces (170g) sugar
- 3.5ounces (99g) walnuts, chopped
- ounces (71g) butter, melted
- 2eggs, lightly beaten
- ¼ teaspoon baking soda

Directions:

1. Select the Bake function and preheat Maxx to 355 degrees Fahrenheit (179 degrees Celsius).
2. In a bowl, combine the sugar, butter, egg, flour, and baking soda with a whisk. Stir in the bananas and walnuts.
3. Transfer the mixture to a greased baking dish. Put the dish in the air fryer oven and bake for 10 minutes.

4. Reduce the temperature to 330 degrees Fahrenheit (166 degrees Celsius) and bake for another 15 minutes. Serve hot.

Nutrition: Calories 70 Total Fat 0.2g Saturated Fat 0.1g Cholesterol 0mg Sodium 1mg Total Carbohydrates 18g Fiber 1.6g Sugar 11.2g Protein 0.6g

Perfect Cinnamon Toast

Preparation Time:10 minutes

Cooking Time: 5 minutes

Servings: 6

Ingredients:

- 2tsp. pepper
- 1 ½ tsp. vanilla extract
- 1 ½ tsp. cinnamon
- ½ C. sweetener of choice
- 1 C. coconut oil
- 12 slices whole wheat bread

Directions:

1. Melt coconut oil and mix with sweetener until dissolved. Mix in remaining Ingredients: minus bread till incorporated.
2. Spread mixture onto bread, covering all area.
3. Pour the coated pieces of bread into the Oven rack/basket. Place the Rack on the middle-shelf of the Air fryer oven. Set temperature to 400 degrees Fahrenheit, and set Time to 5 minutes.

4. Remove and cut diagonally. Enjoy!

Nutrition: Calories 124 Fat 2g Protein 0g Sugar 4g

Apple Pie in Air Fryer

Preparation Time:5 minutes

Cooking Time: 35 minutes

Servings: 4

Ingredients:

- ½ teaspoon vanilla extract
- 1 beaten egg
- 1 large apple, chopped
- 1 Pillsbury Refrigerator pie crust
- 1 tablespoon butter
- 1 tablespoon ground cinnamon
- 1 tablespoon raw sugar
- 2tablespoon sugar
- 2teaspoons lemon juice
- Baking spray

Directions:

1. Lightly grease baking pan of air fryer oven with cooking spray. Spread pie crust on bottom of pan up to the sides.
2. In a bowl, mix vanilla, sugar, cinnamon, lemon juice, and apples. Pour on top of pie crust. Top apples with butter slices.

3. Cover apples with the other pie crust. Pierce with knife the tops of pie.
4. Spread beaten egg on top of crust and sprinkle sugar.
5. Cover with foil.
6. For 25 minutes, cook on 390 degrees Fahrenheit.
7. Remove foil cook for 10 minutes at 330oF until tops are browned.
8. Serve and enjoy.

Nutrition: Calories 372 Fat 19g Protein 4.2g Sugar 5g

Banana Brownies

Preparation Time:5 minutes

Cooking Time: 30 minutes

Servings: 12

Ingredients:

- 2cups almond flour
- 2teaspoons baking powder
- ½ teaspoon baking powder
- ½ teaspoon baking soda
- ½ teaspoon salt
- 1 over-ripe banana
- 3large eggs
- ½ teaspoon stevia powder
- ¼ cup coconut oil
- 1 tablespoon vinegar
- 1/3 cup almond flour
- 1/3 cup cocoa powder

Directions:

1. Preheat the air fryer oven for 5 minutes.
2. Combine all ingredients in a food processor and pulse until well-combined.
3. Pour into a baking dish that will fit in the air fryer.

4. Place in the air fryer basket and cook for 30 minutes at 350 degrees Fahrenheit or if a toothpick inserted in the middle comes out clean.

Nutrition: Calories 75 Fat 6.5g Protein 1.7g Sugar 2g

Chocolate Souffle for Two

Preparation Time:5 minutes

Cooking Time: 14 minutes

Servings: 2

Ingredients:

- 2tbsp. almond flour
- ½ tsp. vanilla
- 3tbsp. sweetener
- 2separated eggs
- ¼ cup melted coconut oil
- 3ounces of semi-sweet chocolate, chopped

Directions:

1. Brush coconut oil and sweetener onto ramekins.
2. Melt coconut oil and chocolate together.
3. Beat egg yolks well, adding vanilla and sweetener. Stir in flour and ensure there are no lumps.
4. Preheat the air fryer oven to 330 degrees Fahrenheit.
5. Whisk egg whites till they reach peak state and fold them into chocolate mixture.

6. Pour batter into ramekins and place into the air fryer oven.

7. Cook 14 minutes.

8. Serve with powdered sugar dusted on top.

Nutrition: Calories 238 Fat 6g Protein 1g Sugar 4g

Blueberry Lemon Muffins

Preparation Time:5 minutes

Cooking Time: 10 minutes

Servings: 12

Ingredients:

- 1 tsp. vanilla
- Juice and zest of 1 lemon
- 2eggs
- 1 cup blueberries
- ½ cup cream
- ¼ cup avocado oil
- ½ cup monk fruit
- 2 ½ cup almond flour

Directions:

1. Mix monk fruit and flour together.
2. In another bowl, mix vanilla, egg, lemon juice, and cream together. Add mixtures together and blend well.
3. Spoon batter into cupcake holders.
4. Place in air fryer oven. Bake 10 minutes at 320 degrees Fahrenheit, checking at 6 minutes to ensure you don't overbake them.

Nutrition: Calories 317 Fat 11g Protein 3g Sugar 5g

Raspberry Cream Roll-Ups

Preparation Time:10 minutes

Cooking Time: 25 minutes

Servings: 4

Ingredients:

- 1 cup of fresh raspberries rinsed and patted dry
- ½ cup of cream cheese softened to room temperature
- ¼ cup of brown sugar
- ¼ cup of sweetened condensed milk
- 1 egg
- 1 teaspoon of corn starch
- 6spring roll wrappers (any brand will do, we like Blue Dragon or Tasty Joy, both available through Target or Walmart, or any large grocery chain)
- ¼ cup of water

Directions :

1. Preparing the ingredients. Cover the basket of the Kalorik Maxx air fryer with a lining of tin foil, leaving the edges uncovered to allow air to circulate through the basket.

Preheat the Kalorik Maxx air fryer to 350 degrees Fahrenheit.

2. In a mixing bowl, combine the cream cheese, brown sugar, condensed milk, cornstarch, and egg. Beat or whip thoroughly, until all ingredients are completely mixed and fluffy, thick and stiff.

3. Spoon even amounts of the creamy filling into each spring roll wrapper, then top each dollop of filling with several raspberries.

4. Roll up the wraps around the creamy raspberry filling, and seal the seams with a few dabs of water.

5. Place each roll on the foil-lined Kalorik Maxx air fryer basket, seams facing down.

6. Air Frying. Set the Kalorik Maxx air fryer Timer to 10 minutes. During cooking, shake the handle of the fryer basket to ensure a nice even surface crisp.

7. After 10 minutes, when the Kalorik Maxx air fryer shuts off, the spring rolls should be golden brown and perfect on the outside, while the raspberries and cream filling will

have cooked together in a glorious fusion. Remove with tongs and serve hot or cold.

Nutrition: Calories 335 Total Fat 15.3g Saturated Fat 8g Cholesterol 28mg Sodium 342mg Total Carbohydrates 45.3g Fiber 0.7g Sugar 30.1g Protein 4.4g

Black and White Brownies

Preparation Time:10 minutes

Cooking Time: 20 minutes

Servings: 8

Ingredients:

- 1 egg
- ¼ cup brown sugar
- 2tablespoons white sugar
- 2tablespoons safflower oil
- 1 teaspoon vanilla
- ¼ cup cocoa powder
- 1/3 cup all-purpose flour
- ¼ cup white chocolate chips
- Nonstick baking spray with flour

Directions:

1. Preparing the ingredients. In a medium bowl, beat the egg with the brown sugar and white sugar. Beat in the oil and vanilla.

2. Add the cocoa powder and flour, and stir just until combined. Fold in the white chocolate chips.

3. Spray a 6-by-6-by-2-inch baking pan with nonstick spray. Spoon the brownie batter into the pan.

4. Air Frying. Bake for 20 minutes or until the brownies are set when lightly touched with a finger. Let cool for 30 minutes before slicing to serve.

Nutrition: Calories 81 Fat 4g Protein 1g Fiber 1g

Baked Apple

Preparation Time:5 minutes

Cooking Time: 20 minutes

Servings: 4

Ingredients:

- ¼ cup water
- ¼ tsp. nutmeg
- ¼ tsp. cinnamon
- 1 ½ tsp. melted ghee
- 2tbsp. raisins
- 2tbsp. chopped walnuts
- 1 medium apple

Directions:

1. Preparing the ingredients. Preheat your air fryer to 350 degrees Fahrenheit.
2. Slice an apple in half and discard some of the flesh from the center.
3. Place into frying pan.
4. Mix remaining ingredients together except water. Spoon mixture to the middle of apple halves.
5. Pour water overfilled apples.

6. Air Frying. Place pan with apple halves into the Kalorik Maxx air fryer, bake 20 minutes.

Nutrition: Calories 199 Fat 9g Protein 1g Sugar 3g

Cinnamon Fried Bananas

Preparation Time:5 minutes

Cooking Time: 10 minutes

Servings: 2-3

Ingredients:

- 1 cup panko breadcrumbs
- 3tbsp. cinnamon
- ½ cup almond flour
- 3egg whites
- 8ripe bananas
- 3tbsp. vegan coconut oil

Directions:

1. Preparing the ingredients. Heat coconut oil and add breadcrumbs. Mix around 2-3 minutes until golden. Pour into bowl.
2. Peel and cut bananas in half. Roll each bananas half into flour, eggs, and crumb mixture.
3. Air Frying. Place into the Kalorik Maxx air fryer. Cook 10 minutes at 280 degrees Fahrenheit.
4. A great addition to a healthy banana split!

Nutrition: Calories 219 Fat 10g Protein 3g Sugar 5g

Awesome Chinese Doughnuts

Preparation Time:10 minutes

Cooking Time: 8 minutes

Servings: 8

Ingredients:

- 1 tbsp. baking powder
- 1tbsps. coconut oil
- ¾ cup of coconut milk
- 6tsps. sugar
- 2cup all-purpose flour
- ½ tsp. sea salt

Directions:

1. Preheat the air fryer to 350 degrees Fahrenheit.
2. Mix baking powder, flour, sugar, and salt in a bowl.
3. Add coconut oil and mix well. Add coconut milk and mix until well combined.
4. Knead dough for 3-4 minutes.
5. Roll dough half inch thick and using cookie cutter cut doughnuts.

6. Place doughnuts in cake pan and brush with oil. Place cake pan in air fryer basket and air fry doughnuts for 5 minutes. Turn doughnuts to other side and air fry for 3 minutes more.

7. Serve and enjoy.

Nutrition: Calories 259 Fat 15.9g Carbohydrates 27g Protein 3.8g

Crispy Bananas

Preparation Time:10 minutes

Cooking Time: 10 minutes

Servings: 4

Ingredients:

- 4 sliced ripe bananas
- 1 egg
- ½ cup breadcrumbs
- 1 ½ tbsps. cinnamon sugar
- 1 tbsp. almond meal
- 1 ½ tbsps. coconut oil
- 1 tbsp. crushed cashew
- ¼ cup corn flour

Directions:

1. Set the pan on fire to heat the coconut oil over medium heat and add breadcrumbs in the pan and stir for 3-4 minutes.
2. Remove pan from heat and transfer breadcrumbs in a bowl.
3. Add almond meal and crush cashew in breadcrumbs and mix well.
4. Dip banana half in corn flour then in egg and finally coat with breadcrumbs.

5. Place coated banana in air fryer basket. Sprinkle with Cinnamon Sugar.

6. Air fry at 350 degrees Fahrenheit/ 176 degrees Celsius for 10 minutes.

7. Serve and enjoy.

Nutrition: Calories 282 Fat 9g Carbohydrates 46g Protein 5g

Air Fried Banana and Walnuts Muffins

Preparation Time:10 minutes

Cooking Time: 10 minutes

Servings: 2

Ingredients:

- ¼ cup flour
- ½ tsp. baking powder
- ¼ cup mashed banana
- ¼ cup butter
- 1 tbsp. chopped walnuts
- ¼ cup oats

Directions:

1. Spray four muffin molds with cooking spray and set aside.
2. In a bowl, mix together mashed bananas, walnuts, sugar, and butter.
3. In another bowl, mix oat flour, and baking powder.
4. Combine the flour mixture to the banana mixture.
5. Pour batter into muffin mold.

6. Place in air fryer basket and cook at 320 degrees Fahrenheit/ 160 degrees Celsius for 10 minutes.

7. Remove muffins from air fryer and allow to cool completely.

8. Serve and enjoy.

Nutrition: Calories 192 Fat 12.3g Carbohydrates 19.4g Protein 1.9g

Nutty Mix

Preparation Time:5 minutes

Cooking Time: 4 minutes

Servings: 6

Ingredients:

- 2cup mix nuts
- 1 tsp. ground cumin
- 1 tsp. chili powder
- 1 tbsp. melted butter
- 1 tsp. salt
- 1 tsp. pepper

Directions:

- Set all ingredients in a large bowl and toss until well coated.
- Preheat the air fryer at 350 degrees Fahrenheit for 5 minutes.
- Add mix nuts in air fryer basket and air fry for 4 minutes. Shake basket halfway through.
- Serve and enjoy.

Nutrition: Calories 316 Fat 29g Carbohydrates 11.3g Protein 7.6g

Vanilla Spiced Souffle

Preparation Time:20 minutes

Cooking Time: 32 minutes

Servings: 6

Ingredients:

- ¼ cup all-purpose flour
- 1 cup whole milk
- 2tsps. vanilla extract
- 1 tsp. cream of tartar
- 1 vanilla bean
- 4egg yolks
- 1-oz. sugar
- ¼ cup softened butter
- ¼ cup sugar
- 5egg whites

Directions:

1. Combine flour and butter in a bowl until the mixture becomes a smooth paste.
2. Set the pan over medium flame to heat the milk. Add sugar and stir until dissolved.
3. Mix in the vanilla bean and bring to a boil.
4. Beat the mixture using a wire whisk as you add the butter and flour mixture.

5. Lower the heat to simmer until thick. Discard the vanilla bean. Turn off the heat.

6. Place them on an ice bath and allow to cool for 10 minutes.

7. Grease 6 ramekins with butter. Sprinkle each with a bit of sugar.

8. Beat the egg yolks in a bowl. Add the vanilla extract and milk mixture. Mix until combined.

9. Whisk together the tartar cream, egg whites, and sugar until it forms medium stiff peaks.

10. Gradually fold egg whites into the soufflé base. Transfer the mixture to the ramekins.

11. Put 3 ramekins in the cooking basket at a Time. Cook for 16 minutes at 330 degrees Fahrenheit. Move to a wire rack for cooling and cook the rest.

12. Sprinkle powdered sugar on top and drizzle with chocolate sauce before serving.

Nutrition: Calories 215 Fat 12.2g Carbohydrates

18.98g Protein 6.66g

Chocolate Cup Cakes

Preparation Time:5 minutes

Cooking Time: 12 minutes

Servings: 6

Ingredients:

- 3eggs
- ¼ cup caster sugar
- ¼ cup cocoa powder
- 1 tsp. baking powder
- 1 cup milk
- ¼ tsp. vanilla essence
- 2cup all-purpose flour
- 4tbsps. butter

Directions:

1. Preheat your Air Fryer to a temperature of 400 degrees Fahrenheit (200 degrees Celsius).
2. Beat eggs with sugar in a bowl until creamy.
3. Add butter and beat again for 1-2 minutes.

4. Now add flour, cocoa powder, milk, baking powder, and vanilla essence, mix with a spatula.

5. Fill ¾ of muffin tins with the mixture and place them into Air Fryer basket.

6. Let cook for 12 minutes.

7. Serve!

Nutrition: Calories 289 Fat 11.5g Carbohydrates 38.94g Protein 8.72g

Air Baked Cheesecake

Preparation Time:20 minutes

Cooking Time: 20 minutes

Servings: 8-12

Ingredients:

- Crust
- 1/2 cup dates, chopped, soaked in water for at least 15 min., soaking liquid reserved
- 1/2 cup walnuts
- 1 cup quick oats
- Filling
- 1/2 cup vanilla almond milk
- 1/4 cup coconut palm sugar
- 1/2 cup coconut flour
- 1 cup cashews, soaked in water for at least 2 hours
- 1 tsp. vanilla extract
- 2tbsp. lemon juice
- 1 to 2 tsp. grated lemon zest
- 1/2 cup fresh berries or 6 figs, sliced
- 1 tbsp. arrowroot powder

Directions:

1. Make the crust: in a food processor, process together all the crust ingredients until smooth and press the mixture into the bottom of a spring form pan.
2. Make the filling: add cashews along with soaking liquid to a blender and process until very smooth; add milk, palm sugar, coconut flour, lemon juice, lemon zest, and vanilla and blend until well combined; add arrowroot and continue blending until mixed and pour into the crust. Smooth the top and cover the spring form pan with foil.
3. Place the pan in your air fry toaster oven and bake at 375 degrees Fahrenheit for 20 minutes.
4. Carefully remove the pan from the fryer and remove the foil; let the cake cool completely and top with fruit to serve.

Nutrition: Calories 423 Fat 3.1g Carbohydrates 33.5g Protein 1.2g

Air Roasted Nuts

Preparation Time:10 minutes

Cooking Time: 20 minutes

Servings: 8

Ingredients:

- 1 cup raw peanuts
- 1/2 teaspoon cayenne pepper
- 3 teaspoons seafood seasoning
- 2 tablespoons olive oil
- salt

Directions:

1. Preheat your air fryer toast oven to 320 degrees Fahrenheit.
2. In a bowl, whisk together cayenne pepper, olive oil, and seafood seasoning; stir in peanuts until well coated.
3. Transfer to the fryer basket and air roast for 10 minutes; toss well and then cook for another 10 minutes.
4. Transfer the peanuts to a dish and season with salt. Let cool before serving.

Nutrition: Calories 193 Fat 17.4g Carbohydrates 4.9g Protein 7.4g

Air Fried White Corn

Preparation Time:10 minutes

Cooking Time: 40 minutes

Servings: 8

Ingredients:

- 2 cups giant white corn
- 3 tablespoons olive oil
- 1-1/2 teaspoons sea salt

Directions:

1. Soak the corn in a bowl of water for at least 8 hours or overnight; drain and spread in a single layer on a baking tray; pat dry with paper towels.
2. Preheat your air fryer toast oven to 400 degrees Fahrenheit.
3. In a bowl, mix corn, olive oil and salt and toss to coat well.
4. Air fry corn in batches in the preheated air fryer toast oven for 20 minutes, shaking the basket halfway through cooking.
5. Let the corn cool for at least 20 minutes or until crisp.

Nutrition: Calories 225 Fat 7.4g Carbohydrates 35.8g

Protein 5.9g

Fruit Cake

Preparation Time:5 minutes

Cooking Time: 45 minutes

Servings: 4-6

Ingredients:

- Dry Ingredients:
- 1/8 teaspoon sea salt
- 1/2 teaspoon baking powder
- 1/2 teaspoon baking soda
- 1/2 teaspoon ground cardamom
- 1-1/4 cup whole wheat flour
- Wet Ingredients:
- 2 tablespoons coconut oil
- 1/2 cup unsweetened nondairy milk
- 2 tablespoons ground flax seeds
- 1/4 cup agave
- 1-1/2 cups water
- Mix-Ins
- 1/2 cup chopped cranberries
- 1 cup chopped pear

Directions:

1. Grease a Bundt pan; set aside.

2. In a mixing, mix all dry ingredients together. In another bowl, combine together the wet Ingredients: whisk the wet Ingredients into the dry until smooth.

3. Fold in the add-ins and spread the mixture into the pan; cover with foil.

4. Place pan in your air fryer toast oven and add water in the bottom and bake at 370 degrees Fahrenheit for 35 minutes.

5. When done, use a toothpick to check for doneness. Of it comes out clean, then the cake is ready, if not, bake for 5-10 more minutes, checking frequently to avoid burning.

6. Remove the cake and let stand for 10 minutes before transferring from the pan.

7. Enjoy!

Nutrition: Calories 309 Fat 27g Carbohydrates 14.7g Protein 22.6g

Hydrated Apples

Preparation Time:5 minutes

Cooking Time: 15 minutes

Servings: 6

Ingredients:

- apples, cored
- 1 teaspoon cinnamon powder
- 1/2 cup sugar
- 1 cup red wine
- 1/4 cup raisins

Directions:

1. Add apples to your air fryer toast oven's pan and then add wine, cinnamon powder, sugar and raisins.
2. Hydrate for 20 minutes and remove from air fry toaster oven.
3. Serve the apples in small serving bowls drizzled with lots of cooking juices.
4. Enjoy!

Nutrition: Calories 229 Fat 0.4g Carbohydrates 53.3g Protein 0.8g

Nutty Slice

Preparation Time:10 minutes

Cooking Time: 30 minutes

Servings: 4

Ingredients:

- 4 cups fresh or frozen mixed berries
- 1 cup almond meal
- 1/2 cup almond butter
- 1 cup oven roasted walnuts, sunflower seeds, pistachios.
- 1/2 tsp. ground cinnamon

Directions:

1. Preheat air fryer toast oven to 375 degrees Fahrenheit.
2. Crush the nuts using a mortar and pestle.
3. In a bowl, combine the nut mix, almond meal, cinnamon and ghee and combine well.
4. In a pie dish, spread half the nut mixture over the bottom of the dish, then top with the berries and finish with the rest of the nut mixture.

5. Bake for 30 minutes. Slice and serve warm with natural vanilla yogurt.

6. Yum!

Nutrition: Calories 278 Fat 15.7g Carbohydrates 10.3g Protein 13.8g

Energy Brownies

Preparation Time: 10 minutes

Cooking Time: 35 minutes

Servings: 10

Ingredients:

- 1-1/2 cups unsweetened shredded coconut
- 1/2 cup dried cranberries
- 1/2 cup golden flax meal
- 1/2 cup coconut butter
- 1 cup hemp seeds
- A good pinch of sea salt

Directions:

1. Combine the cranberries, flax, and hemp seeds in the bowl of your food processor and pulse until well-ground.
2. Add the shredded coconut, coconut butter, stevia, and salt and pulse until it forms thick dough.
3. Transfer the dough to a baking dish and bake for 10 minutes in your air fryer toast oven at 370 degrees Fahrenheit, then remove from air fryer toast oven.

4. Let cool completely, then chill in the fridge to firm up. Slice it into bars and enjoy!

Nutrition: Calories 314 Fat 10.1g Carbohydrates 19.8g Protein 7.8g

Air Fry Toaster Oven Bars

Preparation Time:5 minutes

Cooking Time: 25 minutes

Servings: 4

Ingredients:

- 1 cup chopped chocolate
- 2 ripe avocados
- 1 tsp. raw honey
- 2 tsp. vanilla extract
- 4 eggs
- 1 cup ground almonds
- 1/2 cup cocoa powder
- 1/4 tsp. salt

Directions:

1. Directions: are an 8-inch baking pan by lining it with foil and then coating with non-stick cooking spray.
2. Add chocolate to a bowl and place over a large saucepan of boiling water.
3. Stir until chocolate is melted. Remove from heat and let cool.

4. Meanwhile, Directions: are the batter: in a bowl, mash the avocados; add honey and stir to combine.

5. Whisk in vanilla extract and eggs until well blended. Gradually whisk in the chocolate until well incorporated.

6. Stir in ground almonds, cocoa powder, and salt until well blended.

7. Transfer the batter to the baking pan and cover with a paper towel and then with aluminum foil.

8. Place the pan in your air fryer toast oven and bake at 375 degrees Fahrenheit for 30 minutes or until done to desire.

9. Let cool completely before cutting into squares. These brownies are best served chilled.

Nutrition: Calories 512 Fat 12.3g Carbohydrates 31.2g Protein 14.4g

Self-Saucing Banana Pudding

Preparation Time:5 minutes

Cooking Time: 60 minutes

Servings: 6-8

Ingredients:

- 1 cup caster sugar
- 1 1/2 cups self-rising flour, sifted
- 1/3 cup butter, melted and cooled
- 1 tsp. vanilla extract
- 1/4 cup mashed banana
- 1 egg, lightly beaten
- 3/4 cups milk
- 1/2 cup packed brown sugar
- 1/8 tsp. nutmeg
- 1 tsp. cinnamon
- 1/2 cups boiling water
- ice cream, to serve

Directions:

1. Preheat air fryer oven for 10 minutes.
2. Grease the air fryer oven pan with butter using wax paper.

3. Combine the first 7 Ingredients: above in a large mixing bowl; whisk until well-combined.

4. Fold into the air fryer oven pan. Sift sugar, nutmeg, and cinnamon over the pudding mix.

5. Spoon the boiling water gently and evenly over the mixture.

6. Lock lid in place and cook for 1 hour.

7. Serve hot with a scoop of ice cream on top!

Nutrition: Calories 307 Sodium 76mg Dietary Fiber 0.9g Fat 9g Carbohydrates 54.3g Protein 4g

Chocolate Lava Cake

Preparation Time:5 minutes

Cooking Time: 1 hour 10 minutes

Servings: 6-8

Ingredients:

- 1 box of Devil's Food Chocolate Cake mix, according to box instructions
- 1 (15 oz.) can of milk chocolate frosting, divided
- Non-stick cooking spray

Directions:

1. Spray the air fryer oven pan with cooking spray.
2. Add cake batter as instructed on the box.
3. Spoon half of the chocolate frosting into the middle of the cake batter.
4. Cook for 1 hour.
5. Flip the air fryer oven pan upside down over a cake plate. Heat the remaining frosting in a microwave for 25 seconds, and pour over the warm cake, and serve.

Nutrition: Calories 172 Sodium 91mg Dietary Fiber 0.7g Fat 7.6g Carbohydrates 27g Protein 0.3g

Banana and Walnut Bread

Preparation Time:5 minutes

Cooking Time: 1 hour 10 minutes

Servings: 6-8

Ingredients:

- 1 1/2 cup unbleached flour
- 1/2 cup sugar or sugar substitute
- 2tsp. baking powder
- 1/2 tsp. baking soda
- 1/2 tsp. vanilla extract
- 1/2 tsp. sea salt
- 1 cup ripe bananas, mashed
- 1/3 cup softened butter
- 1/4 cup milk
- 1 egg
- 1/4 cup walnuts chopped

Directions:

1. Combine the flour, sugar, baking powder, baking soda and salt in a large mixing bowl; whisk until the ingredients are well mixed.
2. Fold in the bananas, butter, milk, egg and vanilla extract. Use an electric mixer to mix

until the batter has a uniform thick consistency.

3. Fold in chopped walnuts.
4. Grease the bottom of the air fryer oven pan with non-stick cooking spray.
5. Pour batter into air fryer oven pan and cook for 1 hour. Transfer to plate and let cool for one hour before serving.

Nutrition: Calories 255 Sodium 211mg Dietary Fiber 1.4g Fat 11g Carbohydrates 36.1g Protein 4.6g

Choco-Peanut Mug Cake

Preparation Time:5 minutes

Cooking Time: 20 minutes

Servings: 1

Ingredients:

- 1 tsp Softened butter
- 1 Egg
- 1 tsp butter
- 1 tsp Vanilla extract
- 2tbsps Erythritol
- 2tbsps Unsweetened cocoa powder
- ¼ tsp Baking powder
- 1 tbsp Heavy cream

Directions:

1. Preheat the air fryer for 5 minutes.
2. Combine all ingredients in a mixing bowl.
3. Pour into a greased mug.
4. Set in the air fryer basket and cook for 20 minutes at 400 degrees Fahrenheit

Nutrition: Calories 293 Protein 12.4g Fat 23.3g Carbohydrates 8.5g

Raspberry-Coco Desert

Preparation Time:5 minutes

Cooking Time: 20 minutes

Servings: 12

Ingredients:

- 1 tsp Vanilla bean
- 1 cup Pulsed raspberries
- 1 cup Coconut milk
- 3cups Desiccated coconut
- ¼ cup Coconut oil
- 1/3 cup Erythritol powder

Directions:

1. Preheat the air fryer for 5 minutes.
2. Combine all ingredients in a mixing bowl.
3. Pour into a greased baking dish.
4. Bake in the air fryer for 20 minutes at 375 degrees Fahrenheit.

Nutrition: Calories 132 Protein 1.5g Fat 9.7g Carbohydrates 9.7g

Almond Cherry Bars

Preparation Time:5 minutes

Cooking Time: 35 minutes

Servings: 12

Ingredients:

- 1 tbsp Xanthan gum
- 1 ½ cup Almond flour
- ½ tsp Salt
- 1 cup Pitted fresh cherries
- ½ cup Softened butter
- 2Eggs
- ¼ cup Water
- ½ tsp Vanilla
- 1 cup Erythritol

Directions:

1. Combine almond flour, softened butter, salt, vanilla, eggs, and erythritol in a large bowl until you form a dough.
2. Press the dough in a baking dish that will fit in the air fryer.
3. Set in the air fryer and bake for 10 minutes at 375 degrees Fahrenheit.

4. Meanwhile, mix the cherries, water, and xanthan gum in a bowl.

5. Take the dough out and pour over the cherry mixture.

6. Cook again for 25 minutes more at 375 degrees Fahrenheit in the air fryer.

Nutrition: Calories 99 Protein 1.8g Fat 9.3g Carbohydrates 2.1g

Coffee Flavored Doughnuts

Preparation Time:5 minutes

Cooking Time: 6 minutes

Servings: 6

Ingredients:

- 1 tsp Baking powder
- ½ tsp Salt
- 1 tbsp Sunflower oil
- ¼ cup Coffee
- ¼ cup Coconut sugar
- 1 cup White all-purpose flour
- 2tbsps Aquafaba

Directions:

1. Combine sugar, flour, baking powder, salt in a mixing bowl.
2. In another bowl, combine the aquafaba, sunflower oil, and coffee.
3. Mix to form a dough.
4. Let the dough rest inside the fridge.
5. Preheat the air fryer to 400 degrees Fahrenheit.
6. Knead the dough and create doughnuts.

7. Arrange inside the air fryer in single layer and cook for 6 minutes.

8. Do not shake so that the donut maintains its shape.

Nutrition: Calories 113 Protein 21.6g Fat 2.54g Carbohydrates 20.45g

Simple Strawberry Cobbler

Preparation Time: 10 minutes

Cooking Time: 25 minutes

Servings: 4

Ingredients:

- ¼ cup Heavy whipping cream
- 1 ½ tsps. Cornstarch
- 1 ½ tsps. White sugar
- ½ cup Water
- ¼ tsp Salt
- 2tsps Butter
- 1 ½ cup Hulled strawberries
- 1 ½ tsps. White sugar
- 1 tbsp Diced butter
- 1 tbsp Butter
- ½ cup All-purpose flour
- ¾ tsp Baking powder

Directions:

1. Lightly grease baking pan of air fryer with cooking spray. Add water, cornstarch, and sugar. Cook for 10 minutes 390 degrees Fahrenheit or until hot and thick. Add

strawberries and mix well. Dot tops with 1 tablespoon butter.

2. In a bowl, mix well salt, baking powder, sugar, and flour. Cut in 2 teaspoons butter. Mix in cream. Spoon on top of berries.

3. Cook for 15 minutes at 390 degrees Fahrenheit, until tops are lightly browned.

4. Serve and enjoy.

Nutrition: Calories 255 Protein 2.4g Fat 13g Carbohydrates 32g

Easy Pumpkin Pie

Preparation Time:5 minutes

Cooking Time: 35 minutes

Servings: 8

Ingredients:

- 2Egg yolks
- 1 Large egg
- ½ tsp. Ground ginger
- ½ tsp Fine salt
- 1/8 tsp Chinese 5-spice powder
- 19-inch Unbaked pie crust
- ¼ tsp Freshly grated nutmeg
- 14oz Sweetened condensed milk
- 15oz Pumpkin puree
- 1 tsp Ground cinnamon

Directions:

1. Lightly grease baking pan of air fryer with cooking spray. Press pie crust on bottom of pan, stretching all the way up to the sides of the pan. Pierce all over with fork.

2. In blender, blend well egg, egg yolks, and pumpkin puree. Add Chinese 5-spice powder, nutmeg, salt, ginger, cinnamon,

and condensed milk. Pour on top of pie crust.

3. Cover pan with foil.
4. For 15 minutes, cook on preheated 390 degrees Fahrenheit air fryer.
5. Cook for 20 more minutes at 330 degrees Fahrenheit without the foil until middle is set.
6. Allow to cool in air fryer completely.
7. Serve and enjoy.

Nutrition: Calories 326 Protein 7.6g Fat 14.2g Carbohydrates 41.9g

Simple Cheesecake

Preparation Time:10 minutes

Cooking Time: 19 minutes

Servings: 5

Ingredients:

- 1 cup Crumbled graham crackers
- ½ tsp. Vanilla extract
- 4tbsps. Sugar
- 2 tbsps.   Butter
- 1 lb. Cream cheese
- 2 Eggs

Directions:

1. Mix crackers with the butter in a bowl.
2. Press crackers mixture on the bottom of a lined cake pan.
3. Transfer to the air fryer to cook at 350 degrees Fahrenheit for 4 minutes.
4. Meanwhile, in a bowl, mix eggs, cream cheese, sugar and vanilla, and whisk well.
5. Spread filling over crackers crust and cook in the air fryer at 310 degrees Fahrenheit for 15 minutes.

6. Cool and keep in the refrigerator for 3 hours.

7. Slice and serve.

Nutrition: Calories 245 Protein 3g Fat 12g Carbohydrates 20g

Strawberry Donuts

Preparation Time:10 minutes

Cooking Time: 15 minutes

Servings: 4

Ingredients:

- 4oz Whole milk
- 1 Egg
- 1 tsp. Baking powder
- 1 tbsp. Brown sugar
- 1 tbsp. White sugar
- 8oz. Flour
- ½ tbsps. Butter
- For the strawberry icing:
- 1 tbsp Whipped cream
- ½ tsp Pink coloring
- 2tbsps Butter
- ¼ cup Chopped strawberries

Directions:

1. In a bowl, mix flour, 1 tbsp. white sugar, 1 tbsp. brown sugar and butter, and stir.
2. Stir together the egg with milk, and 1 ½ tbsp. butter in another bowl.

3. Combine the 2 mixtures, stir, then shape
   donuts from this mix.
4. Cook the doughnuts in the air fryer at 3600
   F for 15 minutes.
5. Mix strawberry puree, whipped cream, food
   coloring, icing sugar and 1 tbsp. butter, and
   whisk well.
6. Arrange donuts on a platter and serve with
   strawberry icing on top.

Nutrition: Calories 250 Protein 4g Fat 12g
Carbohydrates 32g

Apricot Blackberry Crumble

Preparation Time:10 minutes

Cooking Time: 20 minutes

Servings: 8

Ingredients:

- 1 cup Flour
- 2tbsps Lemon juice
- 2oz Cubed and deseeded fresh apricots
- ½ cup Sugar
- 2tbsps. Cold butter
- oz Fresh blackberries
- Salt.

Directions:

1. Put the apricots and blackberries in a bowl. Add lemon juice and 2 tablespoons of sugar. Mix until combined. Transfer the mixture to a baking dish.
2. Mix flour, the rest of the sugar, and a pinch of salt in a bowl.
3. Add a tablespoon of cold butter. Combine the mixture until it becomes crumbly. Put

this on top of the fruit mixture and press it down lightly.

4. Move the baking dish in the cooking basket. Cook for 20 minutes at 390 degrees Fahrenheit.

5. Allow to cool before slicing and serving.

Nutrition: Calories 217 Protein 2.3g Fat 7.44g Carbohydrates 36.2g

Ginger Cheesecake

Preparation Time:2 hours 10 minutes

Cooking Time: 20 minutes

Servings: 6

<u>Ingredients:</u>

- ½ tsp. Ground nutmeg
- oz. Soft cream cheese
- 1 tsp. Rum
- ½ cup Crumbled ginger cookies
- ½ tsp. Vanilla extract
- tsps. Melted butter
- Eggs
- ½ cup Sugar

Directions:

- Grease a pan with butter and spread cookie crumbs on the bottom.
- In a bowl, beat cream cheese, eggs, rum, vanilla and nutmeg. Whisk well and spread over the cookie crumbs.
- Place in the air fryer and cook at 340 degrees Fahrenheit for 20 minutes.
- Cool and keep in the refrigerator.
- Slice and serve.

Nutrition: Calories 412 Protein 6g Fat 12g Carbohydrates 20g

Coconut Donuts

Preparation Time: 5 minutes

Cooking Time: 15 minutes

Servings: 4

Ingredients:

- 8ounces coconut flour
- 1 egg, whisked
- 2and ½ tablespoons butter, melted
- 4ounces coconut milk
- 1 teaspoon baking powder

Directions:

1. In a bowl, put all of the ingredients and mix well.
2. Shape donuts from this mix, place them in your air fryer's basket and cook at 370 degrees Fahrenheit for 15 minutes.
3. Serve warm.

Nutrition: Calories 190 Protein 6g Fat 12g Carbohydrates 4g

Blueberry Cream

Preparation Time:4 minutes

Cooking Time: 20 minutes

Servings: 6

Ingredients:

- 2cups blueberries
- Juice of ½ lemon
- 2tablespoons water
- 1 teaspoon vanilla extract
- 2tablespoons swerve

Directions:

1. In a large bowl, put all ingredients and mix well.
2. Divide this into 6 ramekins, put them in the air fryer and cook at 340 degrees Fahrenheit for 20 minutes
3. Cool down and serve.

Nutrition: Calories 123 Protein 3g Fat 2g Carbohydrates 4g

Blackberry Chia Jam

Preparation Time:10 minutes

Cooking Time: 30 minutes

Servings: 12

Ingredients:

- 3cups blackberries
- ¼ cup swerve
- 4tablespoonslemon juice
- 4tablespoonschia seeds

Directions:

1. In a pan that suits the air fryer, combine all the ingredients and toss.
2. Put the pan in the fryer and cook at 300 degrees Fahrenheit for 30 minutes.
3. Divide into cups and serve cold.

Nutrition: Calories 100 Protein 1g Fat 2g Carbohydrates 3g

Mixed Berries Cream

Preparation Time:5 minutes

Cooking Time: 30 minutes

Servings: 6

Ingredients:

- 12ounces blackberries
- 6ounces raspberries
- 12ounces blueberries
- ¾ cup swerve
- 2ounces coconut cream

Directions:

1. In a bowl, put all the ingredients and mix well.
2. Divide this into 6 ramekins, put them in your air fryer and cook at 320 degrees Fahrenheit for 30 minutes.
3. Cool down and serve it.

Nutrition: Calories 100 Protein 2g Fat 1g Carbohydrates 2g

Cinnamon-Spiced Acorn Squash

Preparation Time:5 minutes

Cooking Time: 15 minutes

Servings: 2

Ingredients:

- 1 medium acorn squash, halved crosswise and deseeded
- 1 teaspoon coconut oil
- 1 teaspoon light brown sugar
- Few dashes of ground cinnamon
- Few dashes of ground nutmeg

Directions:

1. On a clean work surface, rub the cut sides of the acorn squash with coconut oil. Scatter with the brown sugar, cinnamon, and nutmeg.
2. Put the squash halves in the air fryer basket, cut-side up.
3. Put in the air fryer basket and cook at 325 degrees Fahrenheit for 15 minutes.
4. When cooking is complete, the squash halves should be just tender when pierced

in the center with a paring knife. Remove from the oven. Rest for 5 to 10 minutes and serve warm.

Nutrition: Calories 172 Protein 3.9g Fat 9.8g Carbohydrates 17.5g

Pear Sauce

Preparation Time:10 minutes

Cooking Time: 15 minutes

Servings: 6

Ingredients:

- 10pears, sliced
- 1 cup apple juice
- 1 1/2 tsp cinnamon
- 1/4 tsp nutmeg

Directions:

1. Put all of the ingredients in the air fryer and stir well.
2. Seal pot and cook on high for 15 minutes.
3. Once done, allow to release pressure naturally for 10 minutes then release remaining using quick release. Remove lid.
4. Blend the pear mixture using an immersion blender until smooth.
5. Serve and enjoy.

Nutrition: Calories 222 Protein 1.3g Fat 0.6g Carbohydrates 58.2g

Brownie Muffins

Preparation Time:10 minutes

Cooking Time: 10 minutes

Servings: 12

Ingredients:

- 1 package Betty Crocker fudge brownie mix
- ¼ cup walnuts, chopped
- 1 egg
- 1/3 cup vegetable oil
- 2teaspoons water

Directions:

1. Grease 12 muffin molds. Set aside.
2. In a bowl, put all ingredients together.
3. Place the mixture into the muffin molds.
4. Press "Power Button" of Air Fry Oven and turn the dial to select the "Air Fry" mode.
5. Press the Time button and again turn the dial to set the cooking Time to 10 minutes.
6. Now push the Temp button and rotate the dial to set the temperature at 300 degrees Fahrenheit.

7. Press the "Start/Pause" button to start.

8. When the unit beeps to show that it is preheated, open the lid.

9. Arrange the muffin molds in "Air Fry Basket" and insert them in the oven.

10. Place the muffin molds onto a wire rack to cool for about 10 minutes.

11. Carefully, invert the muffins onto the wire rack to completely cool before serving.

Nutrition: Calories 168 Protein 2g Fat 8.9g Carbohydrates 20.8g

Chocolate Mug Cake

Preparation Time:7 minutes

Cooking Time: 13 minutes

Servings: 3

Ingredients:

- ½ cup of cocoa powder
- ½ cup stevia powder
- 1 cup coconut cream
- 1 package cream cheese, room temperature
- 1 tbsp. vanilla extract
- 1 tbsp. butter

Directions:

1. Preheat the Smart Air Fryer Oven for 5 minutes at 350 degrees Fahrenheit.
2. In a mixing bowl, combine all the listed Ingredients: using a hand mixer until fluffy.
3. Pour into greased mugs.
4. Place the mugs in the fryer basket and bake for 13 minutes at 350 degrees Fahrenheit.
5. Serve when cool.

Nutrition: Calories 100 Protein 3g Fat 0g Carbohydrates 21g

Chocolate Souffle

Preparation Time:7 minutes

Cooking Time: 12 minutes

Servings: 2

Ingredients:

- 2tbsp. Almond flour
- ½ tsp. vanilla
- 2tbsp. sweetener
- 2separated eggs
- ¼ cups melted coconut oil
- 2oz. of semi-sweet chocolate, chopped

Directions:

1. Preheat the Smart Air Fryer Oven to 330 degrees Fahrenheit.
2. Brush coconut oil and sweetener onto ramekins.
3. Melt coconut oil and chocolate together.
4. Beat egg yolks well, adding vanilla and sweetener.
5. Stir in flour and ensure there are no lumps.
6. Whisk egg whites till they reach peak state and fold them into chocolate mixture.

7. Pour batter into ramekins and place into the Smart Air Fryer Oven, then cook for 12 minutes.

8. Serve with powdered sugar dusted on top.

Nutrition: Calories 378 Protein 4g Fat 9g Carbohydrates 5g

Chocolate Cake

Preparation Time:6 minutes

Cooking Time: 35 minutes

Servings: 9

Ingredients:

- ½cups hot water
- 1 tsp. vanilla
- ¼ cups olive oil
- ½ cups almond milk
- 1 egg
- ½ tsp. Salt
- ¾ tsp. Baking soda
- ¾ tsp. baking powder
- ½ cups unsweetened cocoa powder
- 2cups almond flour
- 1 cup brown sugar

Directions:

1. Preheat your Smart Air Fryer Oven to 356 degrees Fahrenheit.
2. Stir all dry ingredients together and then stir in wet ingredients.
3. Add hot water last.
4. The batter should be thin.

5. Pour cake batter into a pan that fits into the fryer.
6. Bake for 35 minutes.

Nutrition: Calories 378 Protein 4g Fat 9g Carbohydrates 5g

Chocolate Chip Air Fryer Cookies

Preparation Time:10 minutes

Cooking Time: 16 minutes

Servings: 3

Ingredients:

- 75g Self-Rising Flour
- 100g Butter
- 75g Brown Sugar
- 75g Milk Chocolate
- 30 milliliters Honey
- 30 milliliters Whole Milk

Directions:

1. Beat the butter until smooth and fluffy. Add the butter to the sugar and beat together in a smooth mixture. Now add and mix in the milk, sugar, chocolate (broken into small chunks/chips), and flour. Preheat your air fryer to 360 degrees Fahrenheit. Shape the mixture into cookie shapes and put them on a baking sheet that will sit 16 minutes or until cooked through in the air fryer Bake.

Nutrition: Calories 515 Protein 4g Fat 9g

Carbohydrates 5g

Doughnuts

Preparation Time:35 minutes

Cooking Time: 60 minutes

Servings: 8

Ingredients:

- 1/4 cup warm water, warmed (100 degrees Fahrenheit to 110 degrees Fahrenheit)
- 1 tablespoon active yeast
- 1/4 cup, plus half tsp. Granulated Sugar, divided
- 2cups (about 8 1/2 oz.) all-purpose flour
- 1/4 teaspoon kosher salt
- 1/4 cup whole milk, at room temperature
- 2tablespoons unsalted butter, melted
- 1 large egg, beaten
- 1 cup (about 4 oz.) powdered sugar
- 4teaspoons tap water

Directions:

1. Mix water, yeast, and 1/2 teaspoon of the granulated sugar in a small bowl; let stand until foamy, around five minutes. Combine flour, salt, and remaining 1/4 cup granulated sugar in a medium bowl. Add

yeast mixture, milk, butter, and egg; stir it with a wooden spoon until a soft dough comes together. Turn dough out onto a lightly floured surface and knead until smooth, 1 to 2 minutes. Switch dough to a lightly greased tub. Cover and let rise in a warm place until doubled in volume, around 1 hour.

2. Turn dough out onto a lightly floured surface. Gently roll to 1/4-inch thickness. Cut out eight doughnuts using a 3-inch round cutter and a 1-inch round cutter to delete core: place doughnuts and doughnuts holes on a lightly floured surface. Cover loosely with plastic wrap and let stand for about 30 minutes, until doubled in volume.

3. Place two doughnuts and two doughnuts' holes in a single layer in an air fryer pan, and cook at 350 degrees Fahrenheit until golden brown, 4 to 5 minutes. Continue with doughnuts and holes remaining on.

4. Whisk powdered sugar together and tap water until smooth in a medium bowl. In a

glaze, dip doughnuts and doughnut holes, place them on a wire rack set above a rimmed baking sheet to allow excess glaze to drip off. Let stand for about 10 minutes, until the glaze hardens.

Nutrition: Calories 378 Protein 4g Fat 9g Carbohydrates 5g

Cherry-Choco Bars

Preparation Time:7 minutes

Cooking Time: 15 minutes

Servings: 8

Ingredients:

- ¼ tsp. salt
- ½ cup almonds, sliced
- ½ cup chia seeds
- ½ cup dark chocolate, chopped
- ½ cup dried cherries, chopped
- ½ cup prunes, pureed
- ½ cup quinoa, cooked
- ¾ cup almond butter
- 1/3 cup honey
- 2cups oats
- 2tbsp. coconut oil

Directions:

1. Preheat the Kalorik Maxx Air Fryer Oven to 375 degrees Fahrenheit.
2. In a bowl, combine the oats, quinoa, chia seeds, almond, cherries, and chocolate.
3. In a saucepan, heat the almond butter, honey, and coconut oil.

4. Pour the butter mixture over the dry mix, then add salt and prunes and mix until well combined.
5. Pour over a baking dish that can fit inside the air fryer.
6. Bake for 15 minutes.
7. Let it cool before slicing into bars.

Nutrition: Calories 378 Protein 4g Fat 9g Carbohydrates 5g

Crusty Apple Hand Pies

Preparation Time:7 minutes

Cooking Time: 8 minutes

Servings: 6

Ingredients:

- 15-oz. no-sugar-added apple pie filling
- 1 store-bought crust

Directions:

1. Lay out pie crust and slice into equal-sized squares.
2. Place 2 tbsp. filling into each square and seal crust with a fork
3. Pour into the Oven rack/basket.
4. Place the Rack on the middle-shelf of the Smart Air Fryer Oven.
5. Set temperature to 390 degrees Fahrenheit and set Time to 8 minutes until golden in color.

Nutrition: Calories 378 Protein 4g Fat 9g Carbohydrates 5g

Pancakes Nutella-Stuffed

Preparation Time:15 minutes

Cooking Time: 20 minutes

Servings: 12

Ingredients:

- 4teaspoons of chocolate-hazelnut spread, such as Nutella ®, at room temperature
- 1/4 cup vegetable oil, plus
- 1/4 cup grid all-purpose flour
- 1 1/4 cup buttermilk
- 1/4 cup of granulated sugar
- 1 teaspoon baking soda
- 1 teaspoon baking soda
- 1 egg
- A pinch of salt
- Sugar for dusting
- Maple syrup for serving

Directions:

1. Line a parchment baking sheet and drop 12 different teaspoonful mounds of chocolate-hazelnut spread over it. Place the baking sheet on a counter to flatten the dollops and freeze for about 15 minutes until firm.

2. In the meantime, preheat a griddle over low heat and brush with oil lightly.

3. In a large bowl, whisk together the flour, buttermilk, oil, granulated sugar, baking powder, baking soda, egg, and a pinch of salt until smooth.

4. Pour batter pools on the hot griddle and cook until bubbles just start forming on the pancake's surface and the bottoms are golden, 1 to 2 minutes. Place a frozen chocolate-hazelnut dish spread on 4 of the pancakes and flip the remaining four pancakes on top of those, so the wet batter envelopes the disks. Put the rest of the discs back into the freezer. Continue cooking the pancakes for about 1 minute, flipping halfway, until the edges are set. Repeat with the remaining batters and disks, oiling the grid lightly in between lots.

5. Stub the pancakes with the sugar of the confectioners and serve warmly with syrup.

Nutrition: Calories 151 Protein 4g Fat 9g Carbohydrates 5g

Spiced Pear Sauce

Preparation Time:10 minutes

Cooking Time: 6 hours

Servings: 12

Ingredients:

- 8 pears, cored and diced
- 1/2 tsp ground cinnamon
- 1/4 tsp ground nutmeg
- 1/4 tsp ground cardamom
- 1 cup of water

Directions:

1. Put all of the ingredients in the air fryer and stir well.
2. Seal the pot with a lid and select slow cook mode and cook on low for 6 hours.
3. Mash the sauce using a potato masher.
4. Pour into the container and store.

Nutrition: Calories 81 Protein 0.5g Fat 0.2g Carbohydrates 21.4g

Saucy Fried Bananas

Preparation Time: 7 minutes

Cooking Time: 10 minutes

Servings: 2

Ingredients:

- 1 large egg
- ¼ cup cornstarch
- ¼ cup plain breadcrumbs
- 2 bananas, halved crosswise
- Cooking oil
- Chocolate sauce

Directions:

1. Preheat your Kalorik Maxx Air Fryer Oven to 350 degrees Fahrenheit.
2. In a small bowl, beat the egg.
3. In another bowl, place the cornstarch.
4. Place the breadcrumbs in a different bowl.
5. Dip the bananas in the cornstarch, then the egg, and then the breadcrumbs.
6. Spray the basket with cooking oil. Place the bananas in the basket and spray them with cooking oil.
7. Cook for 5 minutes.

8. Open the air fryer and flip the bananas then cook for an additional 2 minutes.

9. Transfer the bananas to plates.

10. Drizzle the chocolate sauce over the bananas and serve.

Nutrition: Calories 378 Protein 4g Fat 9g Carbohydrates 5g

Macaroons

Preparation Time: 10 minutes

Cooking Time: 8 minutes

servings: 20

Ingredients:

- 2 tbsp. Sugar
- 2 cup coconut, shredded
- 4 egg whites
- 1 tsp. Vanilla extract

Directions:

1. In a bowl mix egg whites with stevia and beat using your mixer
2. Add coconut and vanilla extract, whisk again, shape small balls out of this mix, introduce them in your air fryer and cook at 340 °f for 8 minutes.
3. Serve macaroons cold

Nutrition: Calories 55 fats: 6 g carbs 2 g proteins 1 g

Orange Cake

Preparation Time:10 minutes

Cooking Time:16 minutes

servings: 12

Ingredients:

- 1 orange, peeled and cut into quarters
- 1 tsp. Vanilla extract
- 6 eggs
- 2 tbsp. Orange zest
- 4 oz. Cream cheese
- 1 tsp. Baking powder
- 9 oz. Flour
- 2 oz. Sugar+ 2 tbsp.
- 4 oz. Yogurt

Directions:

1. In your food processor, pulse orange very well
2. Add flour, 2 tbsp. Sugar, eggs, baking powder, vanilla extract and pulse well again.
3. Transfer this into 2 spring form pans, introduce each in your fryer and cook at 330 °f, for 16 minutes

4. Mix cream cheese with orange zest, yogurt and the rest of the sugar and stir well.

5. Add half of the cream cheese mix, add the other cake layer and top with the rest of the cream cheese mix.

6. Spread it well, slice and serve.

Nutrition: Calories 200 fats: 13 g carbs 9 g proteins 8 g

Carrot Cake

Preparation Time:10 minutes

Cooking Time:45 minutes

servings: 6

Ingredients:

- 5 oz. Flour
- 3/4 tsp. Baking powder
- 1/4 tsp. Nutmeg
- ground
- 1/2 tsp. Baking soda
- 1/2 tsp. Cinnamon powder
- 1/2 cup sugar
- 1/3 cup carrots, grated
- 1/3 cup pecans, toasted and chopped.
- 1/4 cup pineapple juice
- 1/2 tsp. Allspice
- 1 egg
- 3 tbsp. Yogurt
- 4 tbsp. Sunflower oil
- 1/3 cup coconut flakes; shredded
- Cooking spray

Directions:

1. In a bowl mix flour with baking soda and powder, salt, allspice, cinnamon and nutmeg and stir.
2. In another bowl, mix egg with yogurt, sugar, pineapple juice, oil, carrots, pecans and coconut flakes and stir well
3. Combine the two mixtures and stir well, pour this into a spring form pan that fits your air fryer which you've greased with some cooking spray, transfer to your air fryer and cook on 320 °f for 45 minutes.
4. Leave cake to cool down, then cut and serve it.

Nutrition: Calories 200 fats: 6 g carbs, 22 g proteins 4 g

Perfect Cinnamon Toast

Preparation Time:10 minutes

Cooking Time: 5 minutes

Servings: 6

Ingredients:

- 2 tsp. Pepper
- 1 ½ tsp. Vanilla extract
- 1 ½ tsp. Cinnamon
- ½ c. Sweetener of choice
- 1 c. Coconut oil
- 12 slices whole wheat bread

Directions:

1. Melt coconut oil and mix with sweetener until dissolved. Mix in remaining Ingredients: minus bread till incorporated.
2. Spread mixture onto bread, covering all area.
3. Pour the coated pieces of bread into the oven rack/basket. Place the rack on the middle-shelf of the air fryer oven. Set temperature to 400°f, and set Time to 5 minutes.

4. Remove and cut diagonally. Enjoy!

Nutrition: Calories: 124 Fat:2g protein:0g sugar:4g

www.ingramcontent.com/pod-product-compliance
Lightning Source LLC
Chambersburg PA
CBHW061000050726
47592CB00003B/1285